Sophie B. Nelson

MINDFUL EATING

Savoring the Moment: A Practical Guide to Mindful Eating for Well-Being

Sophie B. Nelson

Acknowledgments

I would like to express my deepest gratitude to the Organization for their invaluable support and guidance throughout the creation of this book. Their wisdom, encouragement, and expertise have been instrumental in shaping this project.

I am also immensely thankful to my family and friends for their unwavering love, understanding, and patience during the writing process. Their belief in me has been a constant source of motivation.

Additionally, I extend my appreciation to the countless authors, researchers, and practitioners whose work has inspired and informed the content of this book. Your contributions to the field of mindful eating have been truly transformative.

Lastly, I dedicate this book to all the readers who embark on this journey with an open mind and a willingness to embrace mindful eating. May it bring you joy, nourishment, and a deeper connection to the present moment.

Sophie B. Nelson

Sophie B. Nelson

TABLE OF CONTENTS

Introduction

Chapter 1: The Foundations of Mindful Eating

Chapter 2: Cultivating Awareness

Chapter 3: Engaging the Senses

Chapter 4: Overcoming Challenges

Conclusion

Acknowledgments

About the author

INTRODUCTION

Introduction: Welcome to Mindful Eating

In today's fast-paced world, where time seems to slip through our fingers like grains of sand, and multitasking has become the norm, it's easy to lose sight of the simple pleasures in life. One such pleasure that often falls victim to our hectic schedules is the act of eating. We rush through meals, barely tasting or appreciating the food that nourishes our bodies, as we juggle work, family, and other responsibilities.

But what if we could reclaim the joy of eating? What if we could transform our relationship with food from one of mindless consumption to one of mindful appreciation? This is where the practice of mindful eating comes in. Mindful eating is not just about what we eat; it's about how we eat, bringing awareness and intention to each bite we take.

At its core, mindful eating is a form of mindfulness—a practice rooted in ancient Buddhist teachings that emphasizes paying attention to the present moment with openness, curiosity, and acceptance. When we apply mindfulness to eating, we become fully present with our food, engaging all of our senses and tuning into our body's hunger and fullness cues. We slow down, savoring each mouthful, and cultivating a deeper appreciation for the nourishment that food provides.

But mindful eating is about more than just the act of eating itself. It's about cultivating a holistic approach to health and well-being—one that encompasses not only what we eat but also how we eat, why we eat, and the broader context in which we consume food. It's about fostering a positive and balanced relationship with food, free from guilt, shame, or restrictive rules.

In this ebook, we will explore the foundations of mindful eating, learn practical techniques for incorporating mindfulness into our eating habits, and discover the many benefits that mindful eating can bring to our lives. Whether you're looking to improve your relationship with food, manage weight more effectively, or simply enjoy a more fulfilling dining experience, the principles and practices outlined in this book can help guide you on your journey toward greater health and happiness.

Throughout these pages, you'll find insights from experts in the fields of mindfulness, nutrition, and psychology, as well as practical exercises and tips to help you integrate mindful eating into your daily routine. Whether you're a seasoned mindfulness practitioner or completely new to the concept, there's something here for everyone.

So, I invite you to join me on this journey of exploration and discovery. Let's slow down, tune in, and savor the moment together as we embark on the path of mindful eating.

Chapter 1: The Foundations of Mindful Eating

Mindful eating is more than just a diet or a trend; it's a way of life—a philosophy that encourages us to bring mindfulness to the dinner table and beyond. In this chapter, we'll delve into the fundamental principles of mindful eating, exploring what it means to eat with awareness and intention.

Understanding Mindful Eating

At its core, mindful eating is about cultivating a deeper awareness of our relationship with food. It's about paying attention to the present moment with curiosity and openness, rather than rushing through meals on autopilot. When we eat mindfully, we engage all of our senses—sight, smell, taste, touch, and even sound—to fully experience the flavors, textures, and aromas of our food.

But mindful eating goes beyond the physical act of eating itself; it also encompasses our thoughts, emotions, and behaviors around food. It involves tuning into our body's hunger and fullness cues, as well as recognizing the emotional triggers that may lead to overeating or unhealthy eating habits. By developing this awareness, we can make more conscious choices about what, when, and how much we eat, ultimately leading to greater satisfaction and well-being.

The Principles of Mindfulness

At the heart of mindful eating lies the practice of mindfulness—a form of meditation that involves paying attention to the present moment without judgment. Mindfulness encourages us to observe our thoughts, feelings, and sensations with kindness and curiosity, rather than getting caught up in them or reacting impulsively.

When applied to eating, mindfulness allows us to become aware of our eating habits and patterns, as well as the thoughts and emotions that arise during meals. By observing these experiences non-judgmentally, we can develop a greater understanding of our relationship with food and make more conscious choices about how we nourish ourselves.

Developing a Mindful Eating Mindset

Cultivating a mindful eating mindset takes time and practice, but it's a journey worth embarking on.

Here are some key principles to keep in mind as you begin your mindful eating practice:

1. Eat with Awareness: Instead of mindlessly devouring your meals in front of the TV or computer, take the time to sit down at the table and savor each bite. Pay attention to the flavors, textures, and sensations of the food, as well as the act of chewing and swallowing.

2. Tune into Your Body: Learn to listen to your body's hunger and fullness cues. Eat when you're hungry, and stop when you're satisfied, rather than relying on external cues like portion sizes or meal times.

3. Eat with Intention: Before each meal, take a moment to pause and reflect on why you're eating. Are you truly hungry, or are you eating out of boredom, stress, or habit? By bringing awareness to your motivations for eating, you can make more mindful choices about what and how much you eat.

4. Practice Non-Judgment: Let go of the urge to label foods as "good" or "bad" and instead approach eating with curiosity and compassion. Notice any judgments or criticisms that arise during meals,

and gently redirect your attention back to the present moment.

5. Cultivate Gratitude: Take a moment to express gratitude for the food on your plate and the nourishment it provides. Recognize the effort that went into growing, preparing, and serving the food, and savor each bite with a sense of appreciation.

By incorporating these principles into your daily life, you can begin to develop a more mindful approach to eating—one that nourishes not only your body but also your mind and spirit.

Chapter 2:
Cultivating Awareness

In the hustle and bustle of daily life, it's easy to fall into the trap of mindless eating—consuming food without really paying attention to what, why, or how much we're eating. But mindful eating invites us to break free from this cycle by cultivating a deeper awareness of our eating habits, thoughts, and emotions. In this chapter, we'll explore how to tune into our body's hunger and fullness cues, identify emotional triggers and eating patterns, and develop a more mindful approach to eating.

Tuning into Your Body's Hunger and Fullness Cues

One of the key principles of mindful eating is learning to listen to your body and respond to its signals of hunger and fullness. This may sound simple, but in a world where we're bombarded with external cues telling us when and what to eat, it can be surprisingly challenging.

To tune into your body's hunger cues, start by checking in with yourself before meals. Ask yourself how hungry you are on a scale from 1 to 10, with 1 being ravenous and 10 being uncomfortably full. Aim to eat when you're at a moderate level of hunger, around a 3 or 4, rather than waiting until you're famished.

During meals, pay attention to the physical sensations of hunger and fullness in your body. Notice the rumbling of your stomach, the sensation of emptiness or fullness, and any other signs that indicate your body's need for nourishment. Eat slowly and mindfully, taking pauses between bites to check in with your hunger levels and assess whether you're still hungry or satisfied.

Similarly, pay attention to your body's signals of fullness. Notice when your hunger begins to diminish and your stomach feels comfortably full. This is your body's way of telling you it's time to stop eating. Trust these signals and honor your body's needs by stopping when you're satisfied, even if there's still food left on your plate.

Identifying Emotional Triggers and Eating Patterns

In addition to physical hunger and fullness cues, mindful eating also involves tuning into the emotional triggers and eating patterns that may influence our food choices and behaviors. Many of us turn to food for comfort, stress relief, or distraction from difficult emotions, leading to mindless or emotional eating.

To cultivate awareness of these emotional triggers, start by keeping a food journal to track your eating habits and the emotions or situations that precede them. Notice any patterns or trends that emerge—for example, do you tend to reach for sweets when you're feeling stressed, or snack mindlessly while watching TV?

Once you've identified your emotional triggers and eating patterns, explore healthier ways to cope with these emotions without turning to food. Practice self-care activities such as meditation, exercise, or spending time in nature to reduce stress and enhance emotional well-being. Develop alternative coping strategies, such as journaling, talking to a friend, or engaging in a creative hobby, to help you navigate difficult emotions without resorting to food.

Developing a More Mindful Approach to Eating

As you cultivate awareness of your body's hunger and fullness cues, as well as your emotional triggers and eating patterns, you'll gradually develop a more mindful approach to eating. Mindful eating is about more than just what you eat—it's about how you eat and the relationship you have with food.

By tuning into your body's signals, honoring your hunger and fullness, and exploring healthier ways to cope with emotions, you can break free from the cycle of mindless eating and cultivate a more balanced and nourishing relationship with food. In the next chapter, we'll explore practical techniques and strategies for incorporating mindfulness into your eating habits, helping you to savor each moment and make more conscious choices about what and how you eat.

Practical Techniques for Cultivating Awareness

Now that we've explored the importance of cultivating awareness in mindful eating, let's delve into some practical techniques and strategies to help you develop this skill further.

1. Mindful Eating Exercises: Practice mindful eating exercises to sharpen your awareness of the eating

experience. For example, try eating a single raisin or piece of fruit mindfully, paying close attention to its texture, flavor, and sensations as you chew and swallow. Notice any thoughts or emotions that arise during the exercise, and observe them with curiosity and non-judgment.

2. Body Scan Meditation: Incorporate body scan meditation into your daily routine to increase awareness of bodily sensations, including hunger and fullness cues. Lie down in a comfortable position and systematically scan each part of your body, from your toes to your head, noticing any areas of tension or discomfort. As you become more attuned to your body's signals, you'll be better able to recognize hunger and fullness sensations during meals.

3. Mindful Eating Journaling: Keep a mindful eating journal to track your eating habits, thoughts, and emotions related to food. Write down what you eat, when you eat, and how you feel before, during, and after meals. Notice any patterns or triggers that influence your eating behavior, and reflect on how you can cultivate greater awareness and mindfulness in your eating habits.

4. Pause Before Eating: Before each meal or snack, take a moment to pause and check in with yourself. Ask yourself how hungry you are and what you're truly craving. Notice any emotional or environmental cues that may be influencing your desire to eat. By taking this pause, you give yourself the opportunity to make a conscious choice about whether and what to eat, rather than reacting impulsively to external cues.

5. Practice Mindful Awareness Throughout the Day*: Extend mindfulness beyond mealtimes by practicing present moment awareness throughout your day. Notice the sights, sounds, and sensations around you as you go about your daily activities. By cultivating a general sense of mindfulness, you'll naturally bring more awareness and intention to your eating habits as well.

Chapter 3:

Engaging the Senses

Eating is a multisensory experience that goes far beyond taste alone. When we engage all of our senses—sight, smell, taste, touch, and even sound—we can fully appreciate the flavors, textures, and aromas of our food, enhancing the eating experience and deepening our connection to the present moment. In this chapter, we'll explore how to harness the power of our senses to cultivate mindfulness and savor each bite with greater awareness and enjoyment.

The Power of Sensory Awareness

Our senses play a crucial role in our perception of food and the eating experience. Each sense provides valuable information about the qualities of food—its appearance, aroma, taste, texture, and even its sound—that can influence our enjoyment and satisfaction with the meal.

Sight: The sense of sight is often the first to be engaged when we encounter food. Take a moment to appreciate the visual appeal of your meals, noticing the colors, shapes, and arrangement of the food on your plate. Pay attention to the vibrant hues of fruits and vegetables, the rich colors of spices and herbs, and the inviting presentation of the dish. By savoring the visual beauty of your food, you can enhance your anticipation and enjoyment of the meal.

Smell: The sense of smell plays a crucial role in our perception of flavor, as it is closely linked to our sense of taste. Before taking a bite, pause to inhale the aroma of your food, allowing the scent to awaken your senses and tantalize your taste buds. Notice the complex aromas that arise from different ingredients and cooking techniques, from the earthy scent of roasted vegetables to the sweet fragrance of freshly baked bread. By paying attention to the smells of your food, you can enhance your appreciation of its flavors and textures.

Taste: Of course, taste is perhaps the most obvious sense involved in eating. But mindful eating invites us to explore taste with greater awareness and intention, savoring each flavor and nuance of the food. Take the time to fully taste each bite, allowing the flavors to linger on your palate and noticing any subtle variations in taste and texture. Experiment with different flavor combinations and seasonings, and pay attention to how they interact to create a harmonious and satisfying eating experience.

Touch: The sense of touch refers to the tactile sensations we experience when handling and eating food. Notice the textures of different foods—crispy, crunchy, creamy, chewy—and how they feel against your tongue and palate. Pay attention to the temperature of the food—whether it's hot, cold, or room temperature—and how it affects your perception of taste and flavor. By tuning into the tactile sensations of eating, you can deepen your connection to the physical experience of nourishing your body.

Sound: Finally, the sense of sound can also influence our perception of food and the eating experience. Listen to the sounds of cooking—sizzling, bubbling, crackling—and the sounds of eating—crunching, chewing, swallowing. Notice how these sounds contribute to the overall sensory experience of the meal, adding another dimension to your enjoyment and appreciation of the food.

Practical Techniques for Engaging the Senses

Now that we've explored the importance of engaging the senses in mindful eating, let's delve into some practical techniques and strategies to help you cultivate sensory awareness and enhance the eating experience:

Mindful Eating Meditation: Practice a mindful eating meditation to focus your attention on each sense as you eat. Take a small piece of food, such as a raisin or a slice of fruit, and examine it closely with your eyes. Inhale deeply to savor the aroma, then place the food in your mouth and chew slowly, paying attention to the taste, texture, and sensation of swallowing. Notice any thoughts or emotions that arise during the meditation, and observe them with curiosity and non-judgment.

Conscious Cooking: Engage your senses in the cooking process by paying attention to the colors, smells, tastes, and textures of the ingredients as you prepare your meals. Take the time to chop, sauté, and season mindfully, savoring each step of the process. Notice how the aromas evolve and intensify as the ingredients cook, and appreciate the sensory pleasure of creating nourishing meals from scratch.

Sensory Exploration: Experiment with different foods and flavors to stimulate your senses and expand your culinary palate. Try incorporating a variety of colors, textures, and aromas into your meals, from vibrant fruits and vegetables to fragrant herbs and spices. Notice how each ingredient contributes to the overall sensory experience of the dish, and be open to discovering new tastes and combinations.

Mindful Dining: Practice mindful eating during meals by turning off distractions such as phones, TVs, and computers, and focusing your attention fully on the food in front of you. Take the time to chew slowly and thoroughly, allowing the flavors to unfold on your palate. Notice any impulses to rush through the meal or reach for seconds out of habit, and gently bring your attention back to the present moment.

Chapter 4:
Overcoming Challenges

While the practice of mindful eating offers numerous benefits, it's not without its challenges. In this chapter, we'll explore some common obstacles to mindful eating and strategies for overcoming them. By addressing these challenges head-on, you can cultivate a more mindful approach to eating and enjoy greater satisfaction and well-being.

Challenge 1: Distractions

One of the biggest obstacles to mindful eating in today's fast-paced world is the prevalence of distractions. From smartphones and TVs to work emails and social media, there are countless distractions vying for our attention during meals. These distractions can pull us away from the present moment, making it difficult to fully engage with our food and eating experience.

Strategy: Create a Distraction-Free Zone

To overcome distractions during meals, create a designated eating space that is free from electronic devices and other distractions. Turn off your phone, TV, and computer, and set aside dedicated time for meals where you can focus solely on the act of eating. By eliminating external distractions, you can cultivate a more mindful eating environment and fully savor the flavors and textures of your food.

Challenge 2: Emotional Eating

Another common challenge to mindful eating is emotional eating—the tendency to turn to food for comfort, stress relief, or distraction from difficult emotions. Emotional eating often involves mindlessly consuming food in response to emotional triggers, rather than eating in response to physical hunger cues.

Strategy: Practice Emotional Awareness

To overcome emotional eating, practice emotional awareness by tuning into your thoughts, feelings, and sensations before, during, and after meals. Notice any emotions or triggers that arise, such as stress, boredom, sadness, or loneliness, and observe them with curiosity and compassion. Instead of turning to food to cope with these emotions, explore healthier ways to address them, such as journaling, talking to a friend, or engaging in a soothing activity like meditation or yoga.

Challenge 3: Cravings

Cravings for certain foods can also pose a challenge to mindful eating, tempting us to indulge in unhealthy or unbalanced foods without regard for our body's hunger and fullness cues. Whether it's a craving for sweets, salty snacks, or rich, indulgent foods, cravings can derail our efforts to eat mindfully and make conscious choices about what we eat.

Strategy: Practice Craving Awareness

To overcome cravings, practice craving awareness by tuning into the sensations and emotions that accompany them. Notice where in your body you feel the craving, whether it's a physical sensation like a rumbling stomach or a mental craving for a specific food. Observe any thoughts or emotions that arise in response to the craving, such as desire, anticipation, or resistance, and allow them to pass without acting on them impulsively. Instead of giving in to the craving, experiment with healthier alternatives or explore the underlying reasons behind the craving, such as hunger, boredom, or emotional distress.

Challenge 4: Time Constraints

In today's busy world, many of us struggle to find the time to eat mindfully amidst our hectic schedules. Whether it's rushing through meals to meet deadlines or grabbing fast food on the go, time constraints can make it challenging to prioritize mindful eating and make conscious choices about what we eat.

Strategy: Make Time for Meals

To overcome time constraints, prioritize making time for meals and set aside dedicated time for eating in your schedule. Even if you have a busy day ahead, carve out at least 15-20 minutes to sit down and eat mindfully, rather than rushing through meals on the run. If time is limited, consider batch cooking or meal prepping ahead of time to ensure you have nourishing meals ready to go when you need them. By making mindful eating a priority, you can reap the benefits of greater satisfaction and well-being, even amidst a busy schedule.

Chapter 5:

Nourishing Your Body and Soul

Mindful eating is not just about fueling your body with nutrients—it's about nourishing your body, mind, and soul with intention and awareness. In this chapter, we'll explore how to make conscious food choices, foster gratitude and appreciation for food, and cultivate a deeper connection to the nourishing power of eating mindfully.

Making Conscious Food Choices

One of the cornerstones of mindful eating is making conscious food choices that support your health and well-being. Rather than mindlessly reaching for whatever is convenient or familiar, take the time to consider how different foods make you feel physically, mentally, and emotionally. Choose foods that energize and nourish your body, rather than leaving you feeling sluggish or unsatisfied.

Strategy: Practice Intuitive Eating

Intuitive eating is a key component of mindful eating that involves tuning into your body's hunger and fullness cues and making food choices based on what your body needs and craves in the moment. Instead of following strict diets or meal plans, listen to your body's signals of hunger and fullness, and trust your instincts to guide you toward foods that satisfy your cravings and nourish your body. By honoring your body's wisdom and intuition, you can develop a more balanced and intuitive approach to eating.

Fostering Gratitude and Appreciation for Food

In our fast-paced, consumer-driven society, it's easy to take food for granted and overlook the many blessings it brings to our lives. But mindful eating invites us to cultivate gratitude and appreciation for the food we eat, recognizing the effort and resources that went into growing, harvesting, preparing, and serving it.

Strategy: Practice Gratitude Rituals

To foster gratitude and appreciation for food, incorporate gratitude rituals into your daily eating routine. Before each meal, take a moment to pause and express gratitude for the food on your plate and the nourishment it provides. Reflect on the journey of the food from farm to table, acknowledging the farmers, producers, and workers who contributed to its creation. By taking the time to cultivate gratitude and appreciation for food, you can deepen your connection to the nourishing power of eating mindfully.

Exploring Mindful Eating Practices

Mindful eating is not a one-size-fits-all approach—it's a personal journey of exploration and discovery that can take many different forms. Whether you're interested in mindful eating for weight management, stress reduction, or simply enjoying a more fulfilling dining experience, there are a variety of mindful eating practices and techniques to explore.

Strategy: Experiment with Mindful Eating Techniques

Experiment with different mindful eating techniques and practices to find what works best for you. Some common techniques include:

Mindful Meal Planning: Plan your meals ahead of time to ensure you have nourishing and balanced options available when hunger strikes. Consider incorporating a variety of colors, textures, and flavors into your meals to stimulate your senses and enhance the eating experience.

Mindful Portion Control: Practice portion control by paying attention to serving sizes and portion sizes, rather than relying on external cues like plate size or portion distortion. Use visual cues such as the size of your hand or a deck of cards to estimate appropriate portion sizes, and listen to your body's hunger and fullness cues to guide your eating.

Mindful Snacking: Snack mindfully by choosing nutrient-dense foods that provide sustained energy and satiety, rather than empty calories or sugary treats. Keep healthy snacks on hand, such as fresh fruit, nuts, seeds, or whole grain crackers, and practice mindful eating techniques such as chewing slowly and savoring each bite.

Chapter 6:
Practical Tips and Techniques

In this chapter, we'll explore practical tips and techniques for incorporating mindfulness into your daily routine. From mindful eating exercises to meditation practices, these strategies can help you cultivate greater awareness and presence in your life, leading to a more fulfilling and satisfying experience.

Mindful Eating Exercises

Mindful eating exercises are a powerful way to deepen your awareness of the eating experience and cultivate a more mindful approach to food. Here are a few exercises you can try:

Mindful Eating Meditation: Set aside time to eat a meal or snack mindfully, focusing your attention fully on the sensory experience of eating. Notice the colors, smells, tastes, textures, and sounds of your food, and savor each bite with curiosity and awareness.

Five Senses Exercise: Engage all five senses in the eating experience by noticing the colors of your food, inhaling its aroma, tasting its flavors, feeling its textures, and listening to the sounds as you chew and swallow. Pay attention to how each sense contributes to your enjoyment and satisfaction with the meal.

Mindful Bites: Take small, deliberate bites of food and chew slowly and thoroughly, paying attention to the sensations in your mouth and throat as you swallow. Notice the flavors and textures of the food, and observe any thoughts or emotions that arise during the eating process.

Meditation Practices

In addition to mindful eating exercises, meditation practices can also help cultivate mindfulness and presence in your daily life. Here are a few meditation techniques you can try:

Breath Awareness Meditation: Sit in a comfortable position and focus your attention on your breath, noticing the sensation of air entering and leaving your nostrils. As thoughts or distractions arise, gently bring your attention back to the breath, without judgment or criticism.

Body Scan Meditation: Lie down in a comfortable position and systematically scan each part of your body, from your toes to your head, noticing any sensations or areas of tension or discomfort. Bring gentle awareness to each part of your body, allowing tension to release and relaxation to deepen with each breath.

Loving-Kindness Meditation: Cultivate feelings of love, compassion, and kindness toward yourself and others by repeating phrases such as "May I be happy, may I be healthy, may I be safe, may I live with ease." Extend these wishes to yourself, loved ones, acquaintances, and even those you may have difficulty with, sending out thoughts of goodwill and compassion to all beings.

Mindful Movement Practices

In addition to seated meditation practices, mindful movement practices such as yoga, tai chi, or qigong can also help cultivate mindfulness and presence in your daily life. These practices involve moving the body with awareness and intention, syncing movement with breath, and connecting mind, body, and spirit.

Yoga: Practice yoga poses or asanas mindfully, focusing your attention on the sensations in your body as you move through each pose. Pay attention to your breath, allowing it to guide your movements and deepen your connection to the present moment.

Tai Chi: Practice tai chi movements mindfully, moving slowly and deliberately with awareness of your body and breath. Notice the sensations of energy flowing through your body as you move, and observe any thoughts or emotions that arise without judgment or attachment.

Qigong: Practice qigong exercises mindfully, focusing on gentle movements and deep breathing to cultivate energy and vitality. Pay attention to the flow of qi or life force energy within your body, and notice how it feels to connect with the universal energy that surrounds you.

Mindful Daily Activities

In addition to formal meditation and movement practices, you can also incorporate mindfulness into your daily activities by bringing awareness and presence to each moment. Here are a few examples:

Mindful Walking: Take a mindful walk outdoors, paying attention to the sensations of your feet touching the ground, the sights and sounds of nature around you, and the rhythm of your breath as you move.

Mindful Washing: Practice mindful washing by bringing awareness to the sensations of water, soap, and movement as you wash your hands or dishes. Notice the temperature and texture of the water, and observe how your hands feel as they move through the washing process.

Mindful Listening: Practice mindful listening by fully engaging your senses in the act of listening to music, nature sounds, or the voice of a loved one. Notice the nuances of sound, from the pitch and rhythm to the emotional tone and resonance, and allow yourself to be fully present with the experience.

Chapter 7:
Mindful Eating in Action

In this chapter, we'll delve into real-life scenarios and practical applications of mindful eating. From navigating social gatherings to eating out at restaurants, we'll explore how to apply mindfulness principles to various situations, empowering you to make conscious choices and enjoy greater satisfaction and well-being in your eating habits.

Mindful Eating at Social Gatherings

Social gatherings often revolve around food, making them both enjoyable and challenging for those practicing mindful eating. Here's how to navigate social events mindfully:

Set Intentions: Before attending a social gathering, set intentions for how you want to approach the event mindfully. Remind yourself of your commitment to listen to your body's hunger and fullness cues, make conscious food choices, and savor each bite with awareness.

Scan the Options: Take a moment to scan the food options available at the gathering, noting which dishes appeal to you and which ones you're less interested in. Choose foods that align with your preferences and dietary needs, and serve yourself small portions to avoid overeating.

Eat Slowly and Mindfully: When it comes time to eat, take small bites and chew slowly, savoring the flavors and textures of each bite. Pay attention to your body's hunger and fullness cues, and pause between bites to check in with yourself and assess whether you're still hungry or satisfied.

Engage in Conversation: Use mealtime as an opportunity to connect with others and engage in meaningful conversation. Focus on the people you're with, rather than getting lost in distractions or mindless eating. Enjoy the social aspect of the gathering and savor the experience of sharing a meal with friends and loved ones.

Mindful Eating at Restaurants

Eating out at restaurants can present unique challenges for mindful eaters, but with a few mindful strategies, you can enjoy dining out while staying true to your intentions:

Review the Menu Mindfully: Take the time to review the menu mindfully, paying attention to the descriptions and ingredients of each dish. Choose options that align with your preferences and dietary needs, and consider asking your server for recommendations if you're unsure.

Practice Portion Control: Restaurant portions are often larger than what we need, so practice portion control by sharing dishes with a dining companion or asking for a half portion. Listen to your body's hunger and fullness cues, and stop eating when you're satisfied, rather than feeling obligated to finish everything on your plate.

Mindful Eating Rituals: Create mindful eating rituals to enhance the dining experience at restaurants. For example, take a moment to express gratitude for the food before eating, or pause to savor each bite with awareness and appreciation. By bringing mindfulness to the dining table, you can deepen your connection to the food and enjoy a more satisfying meal.

Mindful Eating on the Go

In today's fast-paced world, eating on the go is often unavoidable, but with mindful strategies, you can still make conscious food choices and enjoy nourishing meals:

Plan Ahead: Whenever possible, plan ahead and pack healthy snacks or meals to take with you when you're on the go. Choose portable options such as fruit, nuts, seeds, or whole grain crackers, and pack them in a convenient container to enjoy when hunger strikes.

Practice Mindful Snacking: If you find yourself needing to eat on the go, practice mindful snacking by paying attention to the sensations of hunger and fullness in your body. Choose nutrient-dense foods that provide sustained energy and satiety, and eat slowly and with awareness, even if you're in a hurry.

Mindful Fast Food Choices: If you're faced with limited options and need to eat fast food, make mindful choices by opting for healthier options such as salads, grilled proteins, and whole grain options. Avoid supersized portions and sugary beverages, and practice portion control by ordering smaller sizes or sharing with a friend.

Mindful Eating During Stressful Times

During stressful times, it's especially important to practice mindful eating to nourish your body and support your well-being. Here's how to eat mindfully during times of stress:

Check In with Yourself: Before eating, take a moment to check in with yourself and assess how you're feeling emotionally and physically. Notice any signs of stress or tension in your body, and observe any emotions or thoughts that may be influencing your eating behavior.

Choose Comforting Foods Mindfully: If you find yourself turning to food for comfort during times of stress, choose comforting foods mindfully, paying attention to how they make you feel physically and emotionally. Opt for nourishing options that provide comfort without sacrificing your health goals, and practice portion control to avoid overeating.

Practice Self-Compassion: Be gentle with yourself and practice self-compassion during times of stress. If you find yourself turning to food for comfort, acknowledge your feelings without judgment or criticism, and explore healthier ways to cope with stress, such as journaling, talking to a friend, or engaging in a relaxing activity like meditation or yoga.

Chapter 8:

<u>Beyond the Plate</u>

In this final chapter, we'll explore the broader implications and applications of mindful eating beyond the act of nourishing our bodies with food. Mindful eating is not just about what we put on our plates—it's about cultivating a deeper awareness and connection to ourselves, our environment, and the world around us. From fostering gratitude and compassion to promoting sustainability and social justice, mindful eating has the power to transform not only our relationship with food but also our relationship with ourselves and the world.

Fostering Gratitude and Appreciation

Mindful eating invites us to cultivate gratitude and appreciation for the food we eat, recognizing the many blessings it brings to our lives. By acknowledging the effort and resources that went into growing, harvesting, preparing, and serving our food, we can deepen our connection to the nourishing power of eating mindfully.

Gratitude Practices: Incorporate gratitude practices into your daily routine to foster appreciation for the food you eat. Before each meal, take a moment to express gratitude for the food on your plate and the nourishment it provides. Reflect on the journey of the food from farm to table, acknowledging the farmers, producers, and workers who contributed to its creation.

Appreciation for Nature: Mindful eating also encourages us to appreciate the natural world and the interconnectedness of all living beings. Take time to connect with nature through activities such as gardening, hiking, or simply spending time outdoors, and reflect on the beauty and abundance of the earth's bounty.

Cultivating Compassion and Connection

In addition to fostering gratitude and appreciation, mindful eating also promotes compassion and connection—to ourselves, to others, and to the world around us. By cultivating empathy and understanding, we can deepen our connection to ourselves and foster a sense of unity and belonging with all living beings.

Self-Compassion Practices: Practice self-compassion by treating yourself with kindness and understanding, especially when it comes to your relationship with food and eating. Instead of harsh self-criticism or judgment, offer yourself words of encouragement and support, acknowledging that you are doing the best you can in each moment.

Compassion for Others: Extend compassion to others by considering the impact of your food choices on people and communities around the world. Support local farmers and producers, choose ethically sourced and sustainable foods, and advocate for fair labor practices and social justice in the food system.

Promoting Sustainability and Environmental Stewardship

Mindful eating also encourages us to consider the environmental impact of our food choices and promote sustainability and environmental stewardship. By choosing foods that are grown, harvested, and produced in ways that minimize harm to the planet, we can contribute to a healthier and more sustainable food system for future generations.

Sustainable Food Choices: Make sustainable food choices by opting for locally grown and seasonal produce, reducing food waste, and choosing plant-based options whenever possible. Support sustainable farming practices and ethical food production methods, such as organic farming, regenerative agriculture, and fair trade certification.

Environmental Awareness: Stay informed about the environmental impact of food production and consumption, and advocate for policies and initiatives that promote sustainability and conservation. Educate yourself about issues such as climate change, deforestation, and water scarcity, and take action to support initiatives that address these challenges.

Cultivating Mindful Living Beyond the Plate

Finally, mindful eating is just one aspect of a larger practice of mindful living—a way of being present and aware in every moment, both on and off the plate. By cultivating mindfulness in all areas of our lives, we can deepen our connection to ourselves, to others, and to the world around us, leading to greater fulfillment and well-being.

Mindful Movement: Incorporate mindfulness into other areas of your life through practices such as yoga, meditation, tai chi, or qigong. Engage in activities that promote presence and awareness, such as walking, journaling, or spending time in nature.

Mindful Relationships: Cultivate mindful relationships with others by practicing active listening, empathy, and compassion. Be fully present with the people you care about, and cultivate a sense of connection and understanding in your interactions with others.

Mindful Work and Creativity: Bring mindfulness into your work and creative endeavors by approaching tasks with intention and focus. Cultivate a sense of curiosity and openness to new experiences, and allow yourself to fully engage with the creative process, free from judgment or self-criticism.

CONCLUSION

Conclusion: Embracing Mindful Eating as a Way of Life

As we come to the end of this journey exploring the practice of mindful eating, it's important to reflect on the lessons learned and the insights gained along the way. Mindful eating is not just a technique or a diet—it's a way of life, a philosophy that invites us to cultivate greater awareness, presence, and intention in our relationship with food and eating. In this conclusion, we'll summarize key takeaways from our exploration of mindful eating and offer some final reflections on how to embrace mindful eating as a lifelong practice.

Cultivating Awareness and Presence

At its core, mindful eating is about cultivating awareness and presence in the present moment. By paying attention to the sensations, thoughts, and emotions that arise during the eating experience, we can deepen our connection to the nourishing power of food and develop a more balanced and harmonious relationship with eating. Mindful eating encourages us to slow down, tune in, and savor each bite with gratitude and awareness, rather than rushing through meals mindlessly or eating on autopilot.

Listening to the Wisdom of the Body

One of the fundamental principles of mindful eating is listening to the wisdom of the body—tuning into our body's hunger and fullness cues and making food choices based on what our body truly needs and craves in the moment. By honoring our body's signals and eating in response to physical hunger rather than emotional triggers or external cues, we can foster a healthier and more intuitive approach to eating.

Embracing Gratitude and Appreciation

Mindful eating invites us to cultivate gratitude and appreciation for the food we eat, recognizing the many blessings it brings to our lives. By acknowledging the effort and resources that went into growing, harvesting, preparing, and serving our food, we can deepen our connection to the nourishing power of eating mindfully and foster a sense of abundance and gratitude in our lives.

Nourishing Body, Mind, and Soul

Ultimately, mindful eating is about nourishing not only our bodies but also our minds and souls. By approaching eating as a holistic practice that encompasses physical, mental, and emotional well-being, we can cultivate a deeper sense of wholeness and integration in our lives. Mindful eating encourages us to consider the broader implications of our food choices, from their impact on our health and vitality to their effect on the environment and the world around us.

Embracing Mindful Living Beyond the Plate

As we've explored throughout this journey, mindful eating is just one aspect of a larger practice of mindful living—a way of being present and aware in every moment, both on and off the plate. By cultivating mindfulness in all areas of our lives, we can deepen our connection to ourselves, to others, and to the world around us, leading to greater fulfillment and well-being.

Final Reflections

As you continue on your journey of mindful eating and mindful living, remember that it's not about perfection or rigid rules—it's about embracing a spirit of curiosity, openness, and self-compassion as you explore what it means to nourish yourself deeply and authentically. Be patient with yourself, and approach each moment with kindness and gentleness, knowing that every step you take toward greater awareness and presence is a step toward greater well-being and fulfillment.

In closing, may you continue to savor each moment, both on and off the plate, with gratitude, awareness, and joy. May you nourish yourself deeply and authentically, honoring the wisdom of your body and the interconnectedness of all living beings. And may you find peace, joy, and abundance in each moment, knowing that the path of mindful eating is a path of self-discovery, transformation, and growth.

Continuation: Embracing Mindful Eating as a Way of Life

As you continue your journey of embracing mindful eating as a way of life, there are several key practices and principles to keep in mind:

Practice Patience and Persistence

Like any skill or practice, mindful eating takes time and patience to cultivate. Be gentle with yourself as you navigate the ups and downs of the journey, and remember that each moment is an opportunity to start anew. Approach each meal with curiosity and openness, and be willing to learn from your experiences, whether they're moments of success or moments of challenge.

Cultivate Mindful Habits

Incorporate mindful habits into your daily routine to support your journey of mindful eating. Set aside dedicated time for meals, free from distractions, and create a peaceful and inviting eating environment. Practice mindful eating exercises regularly, such as mindful meal planning, mindful snacking, and mindful eating meditations, to deepen your awareness and connection to the eating experience.

Stay Curious and Open-Minded

Approach mindful eating with a spirit of curiosity and open-mindedness, and be willing to explore new ideas and perspectives along the way. Stay curious about your own eating habits and patterns, and be open to experimenting with different mindful eating practices and techniques to see what works best for you. Keep an open mind to the possibility of growth and transformation, knowing that each step you take toward greater mindfulness and presence is a step toward greater well-being and fulfillment.

Foster a Supportive Environment

Surround yourself with a supportive community of friends, family, and fellow practitioners who share your commitment to mindful eating and mindful living. Seek out opportunities for connection and collaboration, whether it's joining a mindful eating group or participating in workshops and retreats focused on mindfulness and wellness. Share your experiences and insights with others, and draw inspiration and encouragement from the collective wisdom of the community.

Reflect and Celebrate Your Progress

Take time to reflect on your journey of mindful eating and celebrate your progress along the way. Notice the shifts and changes in your relationship with food and eating, and acknowledge the moments of growth and insight that have emerged from your practice. Celebrate your successes, no matter how small, and honor the courage and dedication it takes to embark on the path of mindful eating.

Conclusion

In conclusion, embracing mindful eating as a way of life is a journey of self-discovery, transformation, and growth—a journey that invites us to deepen our awareness, presence, and connection to ourselves, to others, and to the world around us. By cultivating mindfulness in our relationship with food and eating, we can nourish ourselves deeply and authentically, honoring the wisdom of our bodies and the interconnectedness of all living beings.

As you continue on your journey of mindful eating, may you find peace, joy, and abundance in each moment, knowing that the path of mindful eating is a path of self-discovery, transformation, and growth. May you savor each bite with gratitude and awareness, and may you nourish yourself deeply and authentically, in body, mind, and soul.

About the Author:

Sophie B. Nelson is a passionate advocate for mindful living and holistic well-being. With over a decade of experience in the field of health and wellness, John has dedicated his career to helping others cultivate greater awareness, presence, and balance in their lives.

Sophie B. Nelson journey into mindfulness began during a period of personal struggle and self-discovery. Faced with the challenges of stress, anxiety, and unhealthy eating habits, he turned to mindfulness as a path to healing and transformation. Through meditation, mindful eating practices, and a commitment to self-care, Sophie B. Nelson experienced profound shifts in his relationship with food and eating, as well as a renewed sense of vitality and well-being.

Inspired by his own journey of transformation, Sophie B. Nelson embarked on a mission to share the teachings of mindfulness with others, believing deeply in its power to enhance every aspect of life. He pursued formal training in mindfulness meditation and mindful eating, studying under renowned teachers and mentors in the field. He became certified as a mindfulness coach and educator, and began leading workshops, retreats, and seminars on mindful living and holistic wellness.

Sophie B. Nelson is known for his compassionate and accessible approach to mindfulness, making the practice accessible to people of all ages and backgrounds. He emphasizes the importance of self-compassion, self-awareness, and self-care in the journey toward greater well-being, and encourages individuals to embrace mindfulness as a way of life, both on and off the meditation cushion.

In addition to his work as a mindfulness coach and educator, Sophie B. Nelson is also a prolific writer and speaker, sharing his insights and wisdom through books, articles, podcasts, and public speaking engagements. He has authored several books on mindfulness, including "The Mindful Path to Wellness" and "Mindful Eating: Nourish Your Body, Mind, and Soul."

Sophie B. Nelson's work has touched the lives of thousands of people around the world, inspiring them to cultivate greater awareness, presence, and balance in their lives. His compassionate and empowering approach to mindfulness has helped countless individuals overcome obstacles, navigate challenges, and discover the transformative power of living mindfully.

In his free time, Sophie B. Nelson enjoys spending time in nature, practicing yoga, and exploring new ways to nourish his body, mind, and soul. He is deeply grateful for the opportunity to share the teachings of mindfulness with others and is committed to supporting individuals on their journey toward greater well-being and fulfillment.

www.ingramcontent.com/pod-product-compliance
Lightning Source LLC
Chambersburg PA
CBHW051704250726
48653CB00007B/2844